The Ultimate Aphrodisiac Cookbook

Everything You Need to Know About Aphrodisiacs

Over 25 Delicious Aphrodisiac Recipes You Can't Resist

BY

Rachael Rayner

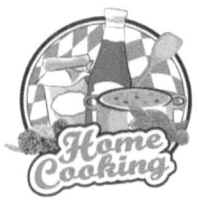

License Notes

No part of this Book can be reproduced in any form or by any means including print, electronic, scanning or photocopying unless prior permission is granted by the author.

All ideas, suggestions and guidelines mentioned here are written for informative purposes. While the author has taken every possible step to ensure accuracy, all readers are advised to follow information at their own risk. The author cannot be held responsible for personal and/or commercial damages in case of misinterpreting and misunderstanding any part of this Book

About The Author

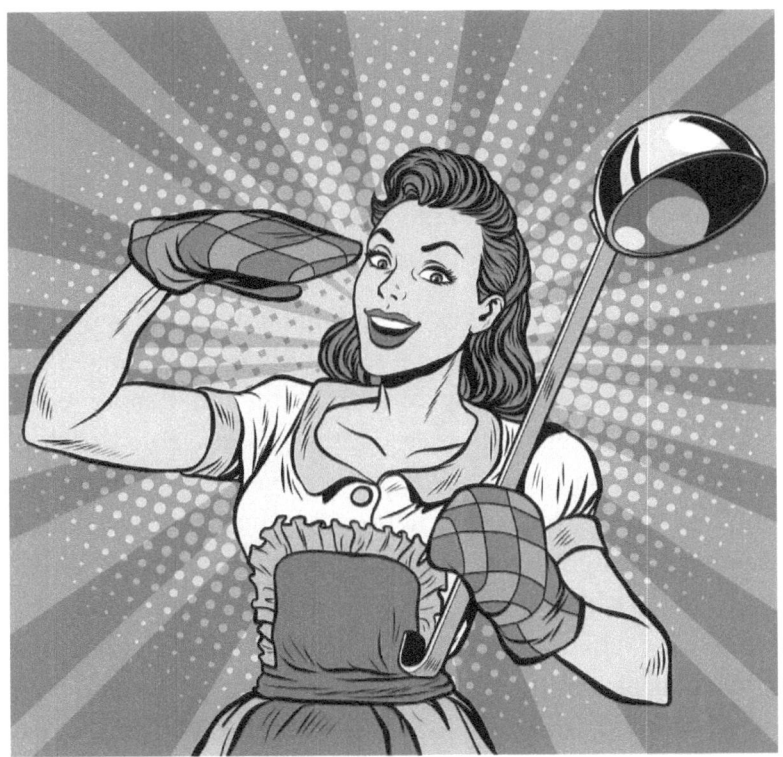

Rachael Rayner

Are you tired of cooking the same types of dishes over and over again? As a mother of not one, but two sets of twins, preparing meals became very challenging, very early on. Not only was it difficult to get enough time in the kitchen to prepare anything other than fried eggs, but I was constantly trying to please 4 little hungry mouths under 5 years old. Of course I would not trade my angels for anything in the world, but I had just about given up on cooking, when I had a genius idea one afternoon while I was napping beside one of my sons. I am so happy and proud to tell you that since then, my kitchen has become my sanctuary and my children have become my helpers. I have transformed my meal preparation, my grocery shopping habits, and my cooking style. I am Racheal Rayner, and I am proud to tell you that I am no longer the boring mom sous-chef people avoid. I am the house in our neighborhood where every kid (and parent) wants to come for dinner.

I was raised Jewish in a very traditional household, and I was not allowed in the kitchen that much. My mother cooked the same recipes day in day out, and salt and pepper were probably the extent of the seasonings we were able to detect in the dishes she made. We did not even know any better until we moved out of the house. My husband, Frank is a foodie. I thought I was too, until I met him. I mean I love food, but who doesn't right? He revolutionized my knowledge about cooking. He used to take over in the kitchen, because after all, we were a modern couple and both of us worked full time jobs. He prepared chilies, soups, chicken casseroles—one more delicious than the last. When I got pregnant with my first set of twins and had to stay home on bed rest, I took over the kitchen and it was a disaster. I tried so hard to find the right ingredients and recipes to make the dishes taste something close to my husband's. However, I hated follow recipes. You don't tell a pregnant woman that her food tastes bad, so Frank and I reluctantly ate the dishes I prepared on week days. Fortunately, he was the weekend chef.

After the birth of my first set of twins, I was too busy to even attempt to cook. Sure, I prepared thousands of bottles of milk and purees, but Frank and I ended up eating take out 4 days out of 5. Then, no break for this mom, I gave birth to my second set of twins only 19 months later! I knew that now it was not just about Frank and I anymore, but it was about these little ones for whom I wanted to cook healthy meals, and I had to learn how to cook.

One afternoon in March, when I got up from that power nap with my boys, I had figured out what I needed to do to improve my cooking skills and stop torturing my family with my bland dishes. I had to let go of everything I had learned, tasted, or seen from my childhood and start over. I spent a week organizing my kitchen, and I equipped myself a new blender. I also got some fun shaped cookie cutters, a rolling pin, wooden spatulas, mixing bowls, fruit cutters, and plenty of plastic storage containers. I was ready.

My oldest twins, Isabella and Sophia are now teenagers, and love to cook with their Mom when they are not too busy talking on the phone. My youngest twins Erick and John, are now 10 years old and so helpful in the kitchen, especially when it's time to make cookies.

Let me start sharing my tips, recipes, and shopping suggestions with you ladies and gentlemen. I did not reinvent the wheel here but I did make my kitchen my own, started storing my favorite baking ingredients, and visiting the fresh produce market more often. I have mastered the principles of slow cooking and chopping veggies ahead of time. I have even embraced the involvement of my little ones in the kitchen with me.

I never want to hear you say that you are too busy to cook some delicious and healthy dishes, because BUSY, is my middle name.

Table of Contents

Introduction

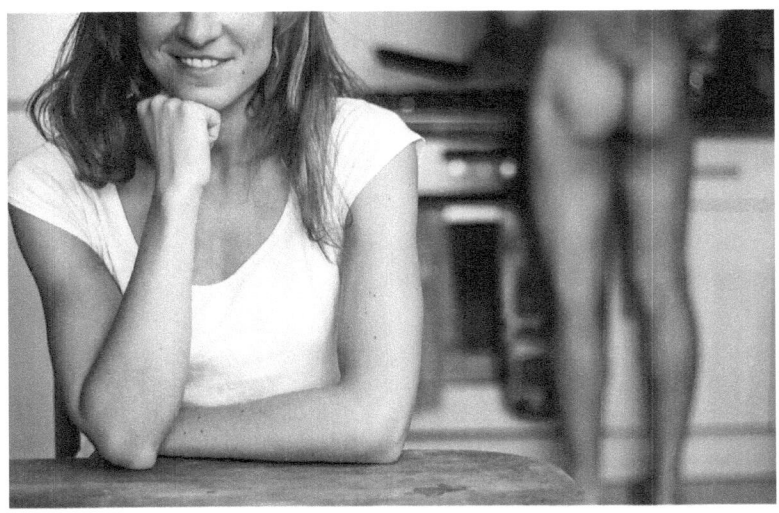

There are many reasons why people want to enjoy aphrodisiacs. Whether you are looking to increase your libido, make your evening with your significant other romantic or simply want to enjoy a delicious meal, you will can enjoy an array of different dishes using these types of ingredients. You name it, you can make it. From tasty oysters to filling salads, you can enjoy aphrodisiacs whenever you wish.

If you have been looking for an aphrodisiac cookbook to make all of your aphrodisiac classics, then this is the perfect book for you. Not only will you learn more about aphrodisiacs in general, but you will also learn about 19 different aphrodisiac foods that you can use as well as discover over 25 different delicious aphrodisiac recipes that I know you will love.

So, let's not waste any more time.

Let's get cooking!

The Benefits of Aphrodisiacs

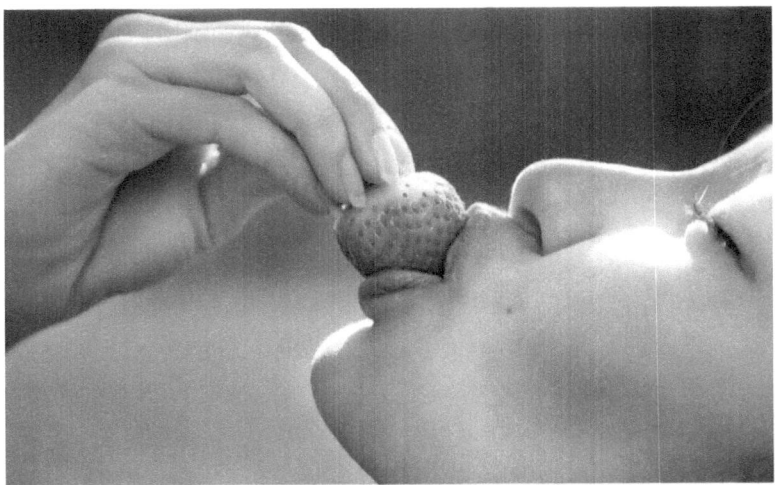

There are various benefits to using and consuming aphrodisiacs other than boosting your libido. So if you have been looking for a list of aphrodisiacs that will help boost the romance in your relationship then this is the perfect section for you. In this section you will learn about the various benefits to consuming aphrodisiacs and how exactly they will benefit your entire body in the long run.

1. Boost Your Memory

There have been many studies conducted that have shown that a few aphrodisiac foods out there such as chocolate can actually help boost your memory. They do this by giving your body extra flavonoids to do so. Not only that but aphrodisiacs such as chocolate can also lower your cholesterol and prevent blood clots as well.

2. High in Nutritious Minerals

We all know that most of the aphrodisiacs that men like to consume tend to be oysters. Oysters have a tendency to have a high reputation because of this. However, these types of aphrodisiacs can also be high in zinc which can also boost the testosterone levels in a man's body. They also contain omega-3 fatty acids which can help protect your eyesight against blindness.

3. Boost Your Red Blood Cell Count

There have been many studies conducted that have found a few aphrodisiacs such as strawberries can also boost the amount of red blood cells currently circulating around your body. With these higher levels of red blood cells in your body it can help increase your energy levels in help fight off anemia. So when your significant other gives you a box full of chocolate covered strawberries, do not turn it down.

4. Increase Testosterone Levels

There are a few different ways that you can increase your testosterone levels naturally by consuming aphrodisiacs. If this is the case the certain foods that you will want to consume are oysters and honey. A study recently conducted in 2001 for the British Medical Journal found when rats were given honey on a daily basis it added more romance to their life.

5. Reduce Mortality Rate

When you often think about aphrodisiacs, the last thing on your mind may be increasing your lifespan. However, when you do just that your life span can be increased. It has been found that by eating aphrodisiacs such as pine nuts you can reduce your mortality rate and can help your live a long and healthy lifestyle. Aphrodisiacs such as pine nuts are also high in manganese which can help aid in overall healthy bone development.

6. Enhance Libido and Control Obesity

Another great benefit of consuming aphrodisiacs on a daily basis is that you can increase both a woman and a man's libido while fighting obesity in the process. When you consume aphrodisiacs such as fennel you can help trick the body into making the production of estrogen in a woman's body which can help fight off obesity.

19 Foods That Are Actually Aphrodisiacs and Can Help Spark Your Romance

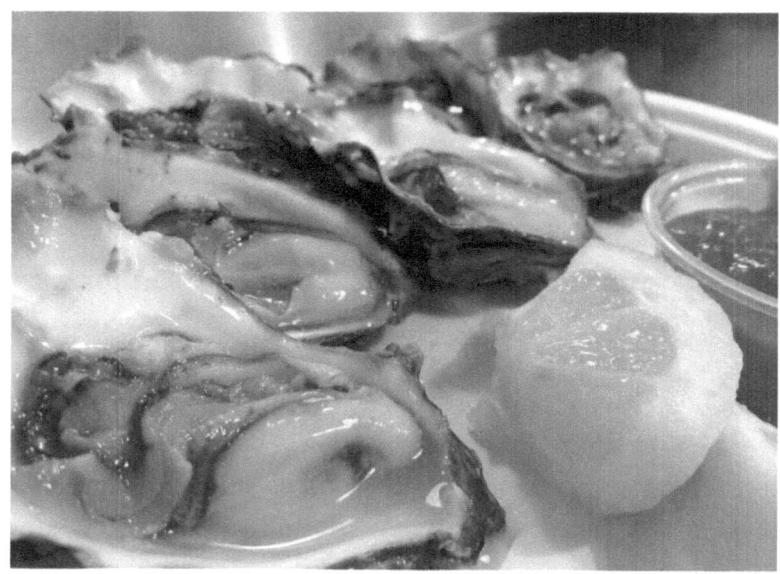

Now that you know how aphrodisiacs can be beneficial for you, and it is time to learn about the different types of aphrodisiacs that you can include into your daily diet. There is no end to the amount of aphrodisiacs available out there and I'm sure after reading this section you will find which ones fit your taste buds the most.

1. Oysters

Oysters seem to be synonymous with aphrodisiacs. Not only are they high in zinc, but they have a great reputation for promoting not only romance but fertility as well. A study recently conducted found that oysters contain amino acids which can help trigger the production of sex hormones in both men and women.

2. Chili Peppers

Chili peppers are not only a great way to spice up your taste buds, but also a great way to add an exotic ingredient into your meal. Chili peppers tend to be a symbol of love as well as an aphrodisiac. However, it has been found that chili peppers can not only stimulate endorphins in your brain, but they can also speed up your heart rate and make you sweat. All of this can be an imitation of how you feel when you are aroused.

3. Avocado

Regardless of whether it is the pear shape or the rich flavor that this fruit has, avocado is another great tasting aphrodisiac that you can enjoy. It has been used as an aphrodisiac since the Aztecs lived on the Earth. This fruit has high levels of vitamin D which can help a person feel young and full of energy.

4. Chocolate

There is just something sensual and great-tasting about chocolate regardless of what color it is. When you consume chocolate it has been shown that it causes a spike of dopamine which is a hormone that acts in your brain and helps to make you feel pleasure.

5. Bananas

Bananas are not only incredibly healthy for you, but they are also a great tasting aphrodisiac as well. Bananas themselves contain an enzyme called bromelain which triggers testosterone to be produced in a man's body as well as help to fuel a body with potassium and vitamin B. These minerals can help increase one's energy levels.

6. Honey

Honey is generally made through the procreation and pollination of bees. Even though it was made out of love honey also contains a compound known as boron which is known to help regulate estrogen and testosterone levels within a person's body. It also has been known to give one heck of an energy boost.

7. Coffee

We all know that coffee can act as a stimulant to help give us energy when we need it in the morning. However, one study has been recently conducted which found that when female rats drink coffee it actually put them in the mood for sex.

8. Watermelon

Surprisingly one study has found that watermelon may be a natural Viagra. It works in the body by relaxing blood vessels and improving circulation which can also enhance arousal in the long run.

9. Pine Nuts

Pine nuts have long been linked to giving a person a healthy sex drive. They are high in zinc which can help boost one's energy, as well as help boost one's performance with their loved one.

10. Arugula

This small peppery plant has been long documented as an aphrodisiac since the very first century. There are many minerals and antioxidants that can be found within the dark leafy greens of this vegetable and it has been known to be able to block contaminants that would actually harm one's libido.

11. Olive Oil

We all know how nutritious and delicious olive oil can be for us. Olive oil is naturally packed with antioxidants and has been used for many centuries because of its ability to promote overall good health. However, olive oil can also make men more virile as well. It has been shown that when olive oil is consumed it can help promote a healthy heart, blood flow and even help to produce hormones.

12. Figs

Figs, the original fruit eaten by Adam and Eve in the Garden of Eden, has been known to symbolize both sexuality and modesty. In real life figs are full of potassium and are one of the powerhouses of antioxidants today.

13. Strawberries

We have already talked about how strawberries can be an aphrodisiac. Strawberries themselves are packed full of healthy vitamin C which can help keep blood flowing through every part of your body. This is essential for an increase in libido.

14. Artichokes

Artichokes have been known as an aphrodisiac for hundreds of years. However, it is a vegetable that is packed full of vitamins and antioxidants which not only help the body to function properly, but also help to keep blood flowing normally as well.

15. Chai Tea

Chai tea is a very delicious drink that many people love to have. When brewed with ginger, cloves and cinnamon, this can help get the blood flowing throughout the entire body without pumping too much harmful caffeine in the process.

16. Pomegranate

This delicious treat is packed full of antioxidants. Antioxidants themselves can help support normal healthy blood flow and has even been found to have a very positive effect on erectile dysfunction.

17. Cherries

Cherries are also known as the world's smallest superfruit. This super fruit is packed full of a variety of different vitamins such as Vitamins A, C and D which are known as the feel good vitamins. It is also packed full of potassium, iron, magnesium, and folate. What is more is that cherries also have melatonin which is an antioxidant that is used to help regulate your heart. This can all lead to a very positive and exciting libido.

18. Pumpkin Seeds

Pumpkin seeds have been proven to be very high in magnesium. In fact, it has at least a 156 milligrams of magnesium in just one ounce of pumpkin seeds. Magnesium has been known to help raise testosterone levels in a male body by making sure more testosterone enters the bloodstream.

19. Whipped Cream

Whipped cream itself tends to be the very image of sensuality. It does not only need to be used as a treat as it can also help increase your libido. While there is no significant evidence to suggest this, you can rest assure that it will put you in the mood in no time.

Delicious Aphrodisiac Recipes

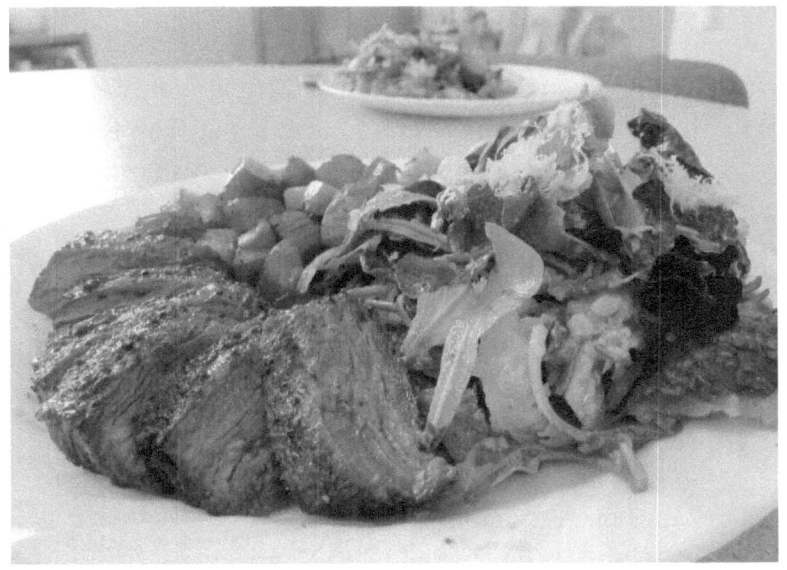

Curry Style Shrimp Salad with Avocado Dressing

Here is a filling and healthy salad recipe that I know you are going to love making over and over again. Top with some creamy avocado dressing to make this dish truly delicious.

Makes: 4 Servings

Total Prep Time: 10 Minutes

Ingredients for Your Avocado Dressing:

- ½ of an Avocado
- ¼ Cup of Yogurt, Plain and Non Fat
- 2 Tbsp. of Vinegar, White in Color
- 3 Tbsp. of Water, Warm
- 1 Lime, Zest Only
- 1 Clove of Garlic, Minced
- 1/8 tsp. of Salt, For Taste

Ingredients for Your Curry and Shrimp Chopped Salad:

- 1 Tbsp. of Olive Oil, Extra Virgin Variety
- 2 Cloves of Garlic, Minced
- ¾ Pound of Shrimp, Raw and Peeled
- 1 tsp. of Curry Powder, Yellow in Color
- ¼ tsp. of Paprika
- Dash of Salt and Pepper, For Taste
- 1 Head of Lettuce, Red Leaf Variety and Roughly Chopped
- 1 Ear of Corn, Fully Cooked and with Kernels Removed
- ½ Cup of Red Onion, Finely Sliced
- 1 Mango, Peeled and Finely Diced

Directions to Make Your Avocado Dressing:

1. First add all of your ingredients for your dressing into a small blender and blend on the highest setting until smooth in consistency.

2. Give your dressing a taste and season with some salt if you wish. Place into your fridge to chill until you are ready to use it.

Directions to Make Your Salad:

1. First add your oil into a large sized skillet placed over medium heat. Once the oil is hot enough add in your garlic and cook for the next 1 to 2 minutes or until fragrant.

2. Next add in your shrimp and continue to cook for an additional minute.

3. Sprinkle with your curry, paprika and dash of salt and pepper, tossing thoroughly to combine. Continue to cook until your shrimp is pink in color and cooked all of the way through. This should take an additional 1 to 2 minutes. Remove and set aside for later use.

4. Next wash and dry your lettuce leaves. Roughly chop them and place into a salad bowl.

5. Then cook your corn in some boiling water for the next 3 to 5 minutes. After this time remove the kernels.

6. Next add your cooked corn and remaining ingredients into your salad and toss thoroughly to combine.

7. Serve with your dressing and top off with your shrimp. Serve right away and enjoy.

Scallops and Black Beluga Caviar Lentils with Microgreens

This is a great tasting aphrodisiac that I know you are going to want to enjoy whenever you get in the mood. It is very delicious to enjoy and for the tastiest results I highly recommend topping this dish with whatever servings you wish.

Make: 2 Servings

Total Prep Time: 40 Minutes

Ingredients:

- 1 Cup of Lentils, Black Beluga Variety
- 4 Cups of Chicken Stock, Homemade Preferable
- 4 Cloves of Garlic, Peeled
- ¼ tsp. of Pepper, For Taste
- 4 Tbsp. of Olive Oil, Extra Virgin Variety
- 4 Scallops, Large in Size
- 1 Egg, White Only and Beaten Lightly
- ½ Cup of Sesame Crust
- 1 Tbsp. of Butter, Soft
- 3 Ounces of Paneer, Cut into Small Sized Cubes
- 2 Cups of Microgreens (Such as Arugula and Cilantro)
- 10 Brussel Sprouts, Shaved
- 4 Radishes, Shaved
- 3 Tbsp. of Cesar Dressing, Your Favorite Kind

- 2 Tbsp. of Relish, Sweet Mango Variety

Directions:

1. First place your lentils, chicken stock, pepper and garlic into a medium sized saucepan placed over high heat.

2. Bring this mixture to a boil before reducing the heat to low. Allow your mixture to simmer for the next 30 minutes or until your lentils are tender to the touch. After this time drain the excess stock.

3. Then puree your garlic cloves with 2 tablespoons of oil in a food processor until smooth in consistency Stir into your lentil mixture.

4. Next pat your scallops dry with paper towels and dip into your egg whites. Roll in your sesame crust and sear in a large sized skillet place over medium heat with some butter for the next 2 minutes on each side.

5. Then use another medium sized pan and heat up your olive oil over medium heat. Once your oil is hot enough and in your paneer and cook until each side is golden in color. This should take about 30 seconds on each side.

6. Toss all of your ingredients together with your micro greens and serve with your dressing. Enjoy.

Chocolate Coffee Rubbed Steak

If you are looking for a fancy dish to make, this is the perfect dish for you. It is quick to put together and one of the most unique steak recipes you will ever come across.

Makes: 2 Servings

Total Prep Time: 20 Minutes

Ingredients:

- 2 Steaks, New York Strip Variety

Ingredients for Your Rub:

- 1 tsp. of Coffee, Ground
- ¼ tsp. of Salt, For Taste
- ¼ tsp. of Garlic, Powdered Variety
- ¼ tsp. of Onion, Powdered Variety
- ½ tsp. of Chili, Powdered Variety
- ½ tsp. of Paprika, Smoked Variety
- 1 tsp. of Cocoa Powder, Unsweetened
- 1 tsp. of Sugar, Coconut Variety
- 1/8 tsp. of Cinnamon, Ground
- Dash of Pepper, For Taste
- 2 Tbsp. of Coconut Flakes, Unsweetened and for Garnishing

Directions:

1. The first thing that you want to do is combine all of your ingredients for your rub in a medium sized bowl until thoroughly mixed. Set aside for later use.

2. Then cut off any visible chunks of fat from your steak and thoroughly coat in your rub. Cover and allow to sit for the next hour to marinate.

3. Next spray a grill pan with a generous amount of cooking spray and preheat over high heat. Then preheat your oven to 400 degrees.

4. Place your steak onto your grill and sear on each side. This should take about 1 to 2 minutes.

5. Reduce the heat to low and continue to cook until your steaks or cook to your desired doneness.

6. Transfer your steak to a plate and cover with aluminum foil. Allow to sit for the next 5 to 7 minutes.

7. Next place your coconut flakes onto a baking sheet lined with parchment paper and toast in your oven for the next 1 to 2 minutes or until golden brown in color.

8. Serve your steak with a garnish of toasted coconut flakes and enjoy.

Spiced Pork with Cherry Sauce

Here is yet another great tasting and easy recipe that you can make whenever you are craving something on the fancier side. It is so delicious I know you won't be able to get enough of it.

Makes: 2 Servings

Total Prep Time: 1 Hour

Ingredients:

- 2 Pounds of Pork Tenderloin
- 2 Tbsp. of Olive Oil, Extra Virgin Variety
- 2/3 Cup of Brown Sugar, Light and Packed
- ¼ Cup of Cocoa Powder, Brown in Color
- ½ tsp. of Paprika
- 1 tsp. of Chili Powder, Ancho Variety
- 1 ½ tsp. of Salt, For Taste
- 1 tsp. of Espresso, Powdered Variety

Ingredients for Your Sauce:

- 2 Tbsp. of Olive Oil, Extra Virgin Variety
- ¼ Cup of Onions, Finely Diced
- ¾ Cup of Cherries, Dried
- 1 Cup of Chicken Broth, Homemade Preferable
- 3 Tbsp. of Vinegar, Balsamic Variety
- 1 tsp. of Rosemary, Dried
- 1 tsp. of Salt, For Taste

Directions:

1. Preheat your oven to 400 degrees. While your oven is heating up spray a baking dish with a generous amount of cooking spray. Set aside for later use.

2. Then rub your olive oil all over your tenderloin.

3. Then use a medium sized bowl and mix together your olive oil, light brown sugar, paprika, espresso, dash of salt, powdered chili and cocoa powder until thoroughly mixed. Rub this mixture onto your pork.

4. Place your pork into your baking dish and place into your oven to bake for the next 45 minutes or until the internal temperature is 145 degrees.

5. Meanwhile make your sauce. To do this heat up your oil in a large sized skillet placed over medium heat. Once the oil is hot enough add in your onions and cook until they are soft to the touch.

6. Then add in your onions, cherries, broth, vinegar, touch of salt and rosemary. Continue to cook until your sauce is reduced by at least half. This should take at least 10 minutes. Remove from heat.

7. After this time serve your tenderloins with your sauce poured over the top. Enjoy.

Seared Duck with Pomegranate

If you have never made duck before, you need to try this recipe out for yourself. This is a delicious dish that makes for the perfect lunch or dinner dish and I guarantee that you won't be able to get enough of it.

Makes: 2 Servings

Total Prep Time: 40 Minutes

Ingredients:

- 2 Duck Breasts
- Dash of Salt and Pepper, For Taste
- 2 Tbsp. of Oil, Grapeseed Variety

Ingredients for Pomegranate Reduction:

- 1, 8 Ounce Bottle of Pomegranate Juice, Pure
- 1 Tbsp. of Maple Syrup, Pure
- Dash of Cinnamon, Ground
- 1/8 tsp. of Salt, For Taste

Directions for Your Pomegranate Reduction:

1. Add all of your ingredients for your pomegranate reduction sauce into a small sized skillet placed over medium heat. Bring it to a boil.

2. Once your mixture has been boiled continue to boil until thick in consistency and reduced by at least a third. This should take at least 30 to 40 minutes.

3. After this time for your pomegranate reduction into a small sized bowl and set aside until ready for use.

Directions for Your Duck Breasts:

1. First preheat your oven to 350 degrees.

2. Cut your meat several times until you make a diamond shape on the surface. Season both sides of your duck with some salt and pepper.

3. Preheat a cast iron skillet over medium to high heat and add just enough oil to coat the surface. Once it is hot enough add in your duck breast and cook for the next 5 minutes or until the skin is brown in color.

4. After this time remove your duck breasts and cover with some aluminum foil. Then place into your oven to bake for the next five minutes.

5. After this time transfer to a cutting board and cut into thin strips.

6. Serve with the drizzling of your pomegranate reduction sauce and enjoy right away.

Pork with Plum and Raspberry Gastrique

Here is yet another great tasting dinner recipe that your significant other is going to love. It is absolutely filling and so delicious, I know you are going to love it.

Makes: 1 Servings

Total Prep Time: 30 Minutes

Ingredients for Your Pork:

- 1 Pork Chop, Large in Size
- ½ Tbsp. of Butter, Soft
- Dash of Mustard, Dried
- Dash of Salt and Pepper, For Taste
- 1 Cup of Broth, Chicken Variety
- 1 Shallot, Fresh
- 1 tsp. of Thyme, Fresh

Ingredients for Your Plum and Raspberry Gastrique:

- 1 Cup of Raspberries, Ripe
- 2 Red Plums, Large in Size, Pitted and Cut into Quarters
- ½ Cup of Vinegar, Red Wine Variety
- 3 Tbsp. of Sugar, Coconut Variety
- Dash of Sea Salt, For Taste

Directions for Your Pork:

1. The first thing that you want to do is add all of your ingredients for your gastrique into a large sized saucepan and cook over medium heat. As it cooks mash everything together with a potato masher and bring to a simmer.

2. Continue to cook for the next 10 to 15 minutes or until thick in consistency.

3. After this time pour through a mesh sieve into a bowl. Return back to your saucepan and season with a touch of salt. Remove from heat and set aside.

Directions for Your Plum and Raspberry Gastrique:

1. Preheat your oven to 400 degrees.

2. Season your pork on both sides with some salt, pepper and mustard.

3. Then use a cast iron skillet and melt your butter into it. Once your butter is melted over medium heat add in your pork and sear on both sides for at least two minutes each side.

4. Continue to cook until your pork reaches your desired likeness.

5. Transfer to your oven to bake for the next 5 to 10 minutes or until completely cooked through.

6. Remove from oven and allow to cool slightly and place onto a serving plate.

7. Then mix together your remaining ingredients in a small size bowl. Drizzle this over your pork along with your sauce and enjoy right away.

Chipotle Style Chicken Stuffed with Goat Cheese

If you are looking for a spicy chicken recipe to enjoy, this is the perfect dish for you to make. This chicken is bold in taste and filled with a spiciness I know you are going to love.

Makes: 2 Servings

Total Prep Time: 30 Minutes

Ingredients:

- 2 Chicken Breasts, Medium in Size
- Dash of Salt and Pepper, For Taste
- 2 to 4 Peppers, Chipotle Variety, in Adobo Sauce and Finely Chopped
- 1 Ounce of Goat Cheese, Crumbled

Directions:

1. First preheat your oven to 400 Degrees. While your oven is heating up grease a baking dish with some non-stick cooking spray and set aside for later use.

2. Next season both sides of your chicken with some salt and pepper and butterfly each breast.

3. Top your chicken with some peppers and goat cheese and fold back over your fillings.

4. Next heat up a large sized skillet placed over medium to high heat. Add in some olive oil and once the oil is hot enough add in your chicken. Sear on all sides until brown in color. This should take at least 5 to 10 minutes.

5. After this time transfer your chicken to your baking dish and place into your oven to bake for the next 15 to 20 minutes.

6. Remove and allow to cool slightly before serving. Enjoy.

Pan Seared Duck Breasts with Orange and Cilantro Sauce

Not only is this yet another mouthwatering duck recipe that I know you are going to love, but it is packed full of the benefits of aphrodisiacs that I know you will love.

Makes: 2 Servings

Total Prep Time: 25 Minutes

Ingredients for Your Orange Sauce:

- 1 ½ Cup of Orange Juice, Freshly Squeezed
- ¾ Cup of Chicken Stock, Homemade Preferable
- ½ Cup of Wine, White in Color
- 1 tsp. of Cilantro, Dried
- 1 tsp. of Parsley, Dried
- ½ tsp. of Black Pepper, Ground and for Taste

Ingredients for Your Duck Breasts:

- 2 Duck Breasts, Fresh
- 1 Shallot, Peeled and Thinly Sliced

Directions:

1. First combine all of your ingredients together for your sauce into a large sized mixing bowl. Stir until thoroughly mixed and set aside.

2. Next you use a sharp knife and score your breasts in a diamond pattern. Season both sides of your duck breast with some salt and pepper.

3. Then heat up a large sized skillet placed over medium to high heat. Once your skillet is hot enough add in your duck breast and cook on both sides until brown and crispy. This should take about 5 minutes on each side.

4. Add in your orange sauce to your pan and continue to cook for the next 10 minutes. After this time remove your duck breast and set aside for later use.

5. Increase the heat to high and allow your sauce to boil until it reduces by at least a third. Remove from heat and serve over your hot and cooked duck breast.

Easy Broiled Halibut with Avocado and Mango Relish

Here is a great tasting fish recipe that every fish lover won't be able to resist. Topped off with delicious and sweet mango and avocado relish, this is one dish I know you are going to want to make over and over again.

Makes: 3 Servings

Total Prep Time: 25 Minutes

Ingredients for Your Halibut:

- 3 Halibut Fillets, ½ Pound Each
- 2 Tbsp. of Oil, Grapeseed Variety
- 1 Lemon, Meyer Variety and Juice Only
- 3 Cloves of Garlic, Minced
- Dash of Sea Salt, For Taste

Ingredients for Your Avocado and Mango Relish:

- 1 Mango, Fresh, Peeled, Pitted and Finely Diced
- ½ of an Avocado, Ripe and Finely Diced
- 3 Stalks of Green Onions, Thinly Sliced
- 1 Lemon, Meyer Variety and Juice Only
- Dash of Salt, For Taste

Ingredients for Your Cauliflower Rice:

- 1 ½ Tbsp. of Oil, Grapeseed Variety
- 2 Cloves of Garlic, Minced
- 1 Head of Cauliflower, Freshly Grated
- ½ tsp. of Cumin, Ground
- Dash of Salt, For Taste

Directions:

1. The first thing that you will want to do this to prepare your mango and avocado relish. To do this add all of your ingredients for your relish into a medium sized bowl and stir thoroughly until mixed. Set aside for later use.

2. Then season your halibut fillets with some salt.

3. Using medium sized bowl and whisk together your grapeseed oil, garlic and lemon juice until thoroughly mixed. Pour over your halibut fillets and allow to marinate for the next 10 minutes.

4. Preheat your oven to broil.

5. Place your fillets into a large sized baking dish and place into your oven to bake for the next eight to ten minutes.

6. Grate the head of your cauliflower using a grater to get your "rice". Add to a large sized skillet with your garlic and cook for the next 3 minutes. Then add in your cumin and salt and continue to cook for at least 8 more minutes.

7. Serve your halibut with your mango relish and cauliflower rice. Enjoy.

The Perfect Roasted Chicken

Just as the name implies this recipe will teach you how to make the most delicious roasted chicken you will ever taste by using a technique that doesn't force you to spend countless hours slaving in your kitchen.

Makes: 4 Servings

Total Prep Time: 55 Minutes

Ingredients:

- 1 Whole Chicken
- Some Olive Oil, Extra Virgin Variety and for Drizzling
- 2 to 4 Tsp. of Your Favorite Herbs

Directions:

1. The first thing that you want to do is preheat your oven to 400 degrees. While your oven is heating up place your baking dish into your oven and allow to warm up as well.

2. Then chop up your whole chicken into small sections and place into a large sized bowl. Add in some olive oil and rub generously with your favorite herbs and spices.

3. Remove your pan from your oven and add in your chicken with the bone side facing down.

4. Place into your oven to cook for the next 20 minutes before flipping the pieces. Then continue to bake for the next 20 to 25 minutes or until the skin of your chicken is golden brown in color.

5. Remove from oven and serve whenever you are ready.

Lamb Lollipops with Mint Pesto

If you are looking for the perfect dish to serve up on Valentine's Day, you can't go wrong with enjoying this recipe. It is incredibly easy to make and so savory, I have no doubt that your significant other is going to love this dish.

Makes: 2 Servings

Total Prep Time: 25 Minutes

Ingredients:

- 1 Rack of Lamb, At Least 6 to 8 Ribs
- 2 Tbsp. of Butter, Soft
- ¼ Cup + 1 Tbsp. of Olive Oil, Extra Virgin Variety
- 1 tsp. of Salt, For Taste
- ½ Cup of Mint Leaves, Fresh
- ½ Cup of Parsley Leaves, Fresh
- 1 Clove of Garlic, Minced
- ½ tsp. of Red Peppers, Crushed
- ¼ Cup of Cashews
- 1 Tbsp. of Vinegar, Rice Variety
- 2 Tbsp. of Water, Warm

Directions:

1. The first thing that you will want to do is combine water, vinegar, cashews, red peppers, parsley, mint, touch of salt and olive oil together in a food processor. Pulse several times until smooth in consistency. Remove and set aside.

2. Then preheat a large sized skillet over medium to high heat. Add in your butter and olive oil.

3. Chop up your lamb and sprinkle with some salt.

4. Place your lamb into your skillet and sear on each side for at least three to five minutes.

5. Next put your pesto into a large sized saucepan and place over medium heat. Allow your pesto to warm gently and add in your butter. Continue cooking until your butter is fully melted. Remove from heat.

6. Serve your lamb onto a serving plate and drizzle your pesto over the top. Enjoy.

Ginger and Orange Glazed Salmon

This is a great tasting meal to make when you are looking for something and easy to prepare on the weekends. It is a low stress and high sex appeal meal that I know you are going to fall in love with.

Makes: 3 Servings

Total Prep Time: 25 Minutes

Ingredients:

- 1 Pound Salmon Fillet
- 1 Tbsp. of Orange, Zest Only
- 1 ½ Tbsp. of Ginger, Fresh, Peeled and Freshly Grated
- 1 Tbsp. of Mustard, Ground
- 1 Clove of Garlic, Peeled and Minced
- 1/3 Cup of Orange Juice, Fresh
- 3 Tbsp. of Olive Oil, Grapeseed Variety
- ¼ tsp. of Salt, For Taste

Directions:

1. Use a small sized bowl and combine your salmon, orange zest, fresh ginger, minced garlic and orange juice together until thoroughly combined. Add in your salmon fillets and toss thoroughly to combine.

2. Place your salmon fillets and marinade into a zip lock bag and allow to marinate overnight or for at least 1 hour.

3. Then preheat your oven to broil.

4. Place your salmon fillets into a large sized dish and drizzle with some olive oil. Season with some salt.

5. Place into your oven to bake for the next 12 to 15 minutes or until your salmon is crispy.

6. Remove and allow to cool slightly before serving.

Classic Orange Chicken

Want a low stress and incredibly delicious recipe to put together? Well, you can't go wrong with this dish. For the tastiest results feel free to serve this dish alongside any side of your choice.

Makes: 2 Servings

Total Prep Time: 25 Minutes

Ingredients for Your Sauce:

- ½ Cup of Sugar, White
- 2 Tbsp. of Vinegar, Rice Variety
- ½ Cup of Orange Juice, Fresh
- 2 Oranges, Zest Only
- 2 to 3 Cloves of Garlic, Freshly Grated
- 2 Tbsp. of Ginger, Fresh, Peeled and Grated
- ¼ tsp. of Sea Salt, For Taste

Ingredients for Your Chicken:

- 2 Chicken Breasts, Boneless and Skinless Variety
- 2 Tbsp. of Oil, Cooking Variety
- Dash of Salt and Pepper, For Taste

Directions to Make Your Sauce:

1. To make your sauce you will first want to heat up your sugar and vinegar in a medium sized saucepan placed over medium heat. Cook until your sugar fully dissolves.

2. Then reduce the heat to low and add in your orange juice and zest. Continue to cook for the next 3 to 4 minutes until simmering. Then add in your grated garlic, sea salt and grated ginger.

3. Continue simmering for the next 10 minutes until your sauce is thick in consistency.

Directions to Make Your Chicken:

1. Then heat up some oil in a large sized skillet place over medium heat.

2. Season your chicken breast with some salt and pepper. Place into your skillet to cook once it was hot enough for the next five minutes. Flip and continue to cook for an additional 5 to 7 more minutes.

3. Then add your sauce into your pan and allow to cook at a simmer for the next 6 to 8 minutes. Make sure that you spoon your sauce continuously over your chicken.

4. When your chicken is fully cooked through remove from heat and serve right away. Enjoy.

Aphrodisiac Olive and Chocolate Love Bombs

If you really want to put yourself in the mood in a relatively quick fashion, then this is the dish you need to prepare for yourself. While I know that olives and chocolates do not sound like the best pairing, you will not think the same once you get a taste.

Makes: 30 Servings

Total Prep Time: 10 Minutes

Ingredients:

- 2 ½ Ounces of Chocolate, Dark in Color
- 20 Olives, Green in Color and Large in Size
- 2 Ounces of Ricotta Cheese, Fresh
- 1 tsp. of Lemon, Zest Only
- 1 Tbsp. of Sugar, White
- ¼ tsp. of Vanilla, Pure

Directions:

1. The first thing that you want to do is melt your dark chocolate in a microwave until fully melted.

2. Then dip the closed end of your green olives into your chocolate at least half way.

3. Place onto a sheet of parchment paper to rest for the next couple of minutes.

4. Melt any of your remaining chocolate with your remaining ingredients until fully melted and evenly combined.

5. Pipe this chocolate filling into your olives. Place into your fridge to chill until you are ready to enjoy them.

Tasty Crab Cakes with Zucchini Noodles

Here is yet another delicious aphrodisiac recipe that I know you are going to love. Not only is it very delicious, but it is also healthy as well. With this dish you do not have to worry about feeling guilty after eating it.

Makes: 2 Servings

Total Prep Time: 45 Minutes

Ingredients:

- 7 Sticks of Crab Meat, Imitation Variety and Chopped Coarsely
- 1 Red Pepper, Small in Size and Finely Diced
- 4 Onions, Green in Color and Finely Diced
- 1 Jalapeno, Finely Diced
- ½ of a Lime, Juice Only
- ½ Cup of Mayonnaise, Your Favorite Kind
- ½ Cup of Matzah Meal
- 1 Bunch of Cilantro, Chopped Roughly
- 1 Tbsp. of Cumin, Ground
- ½ Tbsp. of Salt, For Taste
- ½ Tbsp. of Pepper, For Taste
- 5 Tbsp. of Oil, Cooking Variety
- 1 Zucchini, Large in Size and Sliced into Thin Noodles

Ingredients for Your Avocado Crema:

- ½ Cup of Sour Cream
- ½ Cup of Mayonnaise, Your Favorite Kind
- ½ of an Avocado, Fresh
- 1 Tbsp. of Lime Juice, Fresh

Directions:

1. Use a small sized bowl and whisk your mayo, avocado and lime juice together. Add in your sour cream and continue to mix until thoroughly combined. Set this mixture aside.

2. Then use a large sized bowl and mix together your crab meat with your remaining mayo, meal, peppers, onions, cilantro, cumin, dash of salt and pepper and jalapenos. Stir thoroughly until evenly mixed.

3. Shape your crab mixture into even sized patties and place into your fridge to chill for the next 30 minutes.

4. Then use a large saucepan place over medium heat. Add in your oil and when the oil is hot enough fry your crab cakes until golden brown in color and crispy. This take at least two minutes on each side.

5. Serve your crab cakes on top of a bed of zucchini noodles and dash of your avocado cream. Enjoy whenever you are ready.

Traditional Mussels Fra Diavolo

This is a great dish to make if you are able to get mussels fresh. It is a great dish to enjoy for the average sea lover and is packed full of the benefits of aphrodisiacs that you love.

Makes: 6 Servings

Total Prep Time: 1 Hour and 35 Minutes

Ingredients for Your Sauce:

- 2 Tbsp. of Olive Oil, Extra Virgin Variety
- 2 Bay Leaves, Fresh
- 1 Head of Garlic, Peeled, Smashed and Minced
- 2 Onions, Yellow in Color and Finely Chopped
- 2 Carrots, Medium in Size, Peeled and Finely Chopped
- 1 ½ tsp. of Oregano, Dried
- 1 ½ tsp. of Red Pepper Flakes, Crushed
- 3 Red Chilies, Dried
- 2, 8 Ounce Cans of Tomatoes, Plum Variety, Peeled and Crushed
- 2 Tbsp. of Tomato Paste
- 1, 8 Ounce Bottle of Clam Juice
- ½ Cup of Wine, White in Color
- 2 tsp. of Salt, For Taste
- 1 tsp. of Black Pepper, For Taste
- ½ tsp. of Sugar, Coconut and Palm Variety

Ingredients for Your Mussels:

- 1 Tbsp. of Olive Oil, Extra Virgin Variety
- 3 Shallots, Finely Chopped
- 1 Cup of Wine, White in Color
- 4 Pounds of Mussels, De-Bearded and Cleaned
- 1 Handful of Parsley, Flat Leaf Variety and Roughly Chopped

Directions:

1. First chop up your garlic, onions and carrots.

2. Place for your tomatoes into a large sized bowl and squeeze your tomatoes to gently crush them.

3. Heat up a large sized pot placed over medium to high. Add in your oil and once it is hot enough add in your bay leaves. Cook for at least 30 seconds until sizzling.

4. Then add in your garlic and cook for at least one minute until fragrant. Make sure that you stir your garlic constantly.

5. Then add in your chopped up carrots, onions along with your oregano, chilies and red pepper flakes. Stir thoroughly to combine and allow to cook for the next 15 minutes or until your onions are brown in color.

6. Then add in your crushed tomatoes with the juice along with the remaining ingredients except for your mussels. Allow your mixture to come to a boil. Once your mixture is boiling reduce the heat to low and allow to simmer for the next hour.

7. After this time add in your muscles and allow to cook until they all open by themselves. Toss away any mussels that do not open. Boil for at least 10 more minutes and remove from heat. Serve whenever you are ready.

Drunk Clams and Sausage

This dish is made by using only the highest quality ingredients such as white wine, fennel, fresh clams and sausage, making it the perfect dish to make if you are looking for something homey and filling. For the tastiest results I highly recommend serving this dish with some crusty bread on the side.

Makes: 4 Servings

Total Prep Time: 1 Hour and 35 Minutes

Ingredients:

- 2 Tbsp. of Olive Oil, Extra Virgin Variety
- 1 Pound of Sausage, Italian Variety and Casing Removed
- 2 Shallots, Minced
- 1 Head of Fennel, Medium in Size and Thinly Sliced
- 2 Cloves of Garlic, Minced
- 1 Cup of Wine, White in Color and Dry Variety
- 1 Cup of Chicken Stock, Homemade Preferable and Low in Sodium
- 2 Dozen Clams, Little Neck Variety, Rinsed and Cleaned
- ½ Cup of Cream, Heavy Variety

Directions:

1. Use a large sized skillet placed over medium heat. Add in your oil and once your oil is hot enough add in your sausage and cook until brown in color.

2. Then add in your shallots and fennel and continue to cook until they are soft to the touch.

3. Add in your garlic and continue to cook for an additional minute.

4. Add in your white wine and allow it to continue cooking until reduced by at least half. Then add in your chicken stock. Stir thoroughly to combine.

5. Place your clams on top of this mixture and push them into your stock. Cover and allow to cook for at least 8 minutes or until completely opened. Toss out any clams that do not open.

6. Remove your clams from your mixture and add in your cream. Continue to cook for 5 minutes or until piping hot.

7. Place your clams back into your mixture and remove from heat. Serve whenever you are ready.

Pineapple and Fennel Salad with Sesame and Ginger Dressing

If you have been craving a healthy and delicious salad recipe, then this is certainly the dish for you to make. Feel free to be as creative as you want with this dish. Either way it is going to taste amazing.

Makes: 2 Servings

Total Prep Time: 15 Minutes

Ingredients for Your Dressing:

- 1 ½ Tbsp. of Lemon Juice, Fresh
- 1 Tbsp. of Honey, Raw
- 1 Tbsp. of Sugar
- 2 tsp. of Ginger, Fresh and Grated
- 2 Tbsp. of Oil, Sesame Variety
- 2 Tbsp. of Sesame Seeds, Slightly Toasted

Ingredients for Your Salad:

- 1 Head of Fennel, Medium in Size, Cut into Quarters and Sliced Thinly
- 1 Cup of Pineapple, Fresh and Finely Diced
- 1 Cup of Radishes, Sliced Thinly
- 2 Green Onions, Sliced Thinly
- 1 Cup of Avocado, Finely Diced
- 3 Cups of Arugula, Fresh

Directions:

1. The first thing that you want to do is prepare all of your ingredients for your salad.

2. Then place into a large salad bowl and toss thoroughly until mixed.

3. Make your salad dressing next by mixing together all of your ingredients for dressing with a whisk until smooth in consistency.

4. Pour over your dressing and toss thoroughly to coat. Serve whenever you are ready. Enjoy.

Greens and Blackberry Salad

Here is yet another great tasting salad recipe that I know you are not going to get enough of. For the tastiest results, make sure that you only use the freshest ingredients possible.

Makes: 4 to 6 Servings

Total Prep Time: 20 Minutes

Ingredients for Your Salad:

- 3 Cups of Leafy Greens, Washed, Dried and Torn into Small Pieces
- 1 Pint of Blackberries, Fresh, Washed and Dried
- 2 Green Onions, Sliced Thinly
- ½ Cup of Almonds, Sliced and Lightly Toasted
- ¼ Cup of Goat Cheese, Finely Diced

Ingredients for Your Vinaigrette:

- 1 Tbsp. of Honey, Raw
- ¼ Cup of Vinegar, Blackberry and Ginger Variety
- ¼ Cup of Olive Oil, Extra Virgin Variety
- 1 Green Onion, Minced
- ¼ tsp. of Salt, For Taste
- ¼ tsp. of Black Pepper, For Taste
- 1 Tbsp. of Tarragon, Fresh and Roughly Diced
- 1 Tbsp. of Mint, Fresh and Roughly Chopped

Directions:

1. The first thing that you want to do is mix all of your ingredients for your salad together in a large sized salad bowl. Then cover and place into your refrigerator to chill until you are ready to serve.

2. Then mix all of your ingredients together except for your olive oil for your vinaigrette into a medium sized bowl. Whisk until smooth in consistency and evenly blended.

3. As you are mixing gently drizzle in your olive oil and continue mixing until evenly incorporated.

4. Serve your salad with a drizzling of your fresh homemade salad dressing over the top and enjoy right away.

Delicious Caramelized Brussels Sprouts

Here is a tasty side dish that I know you are going to want to serve with every dinner dish that you make. The citrus flavor helps to add a touch of sweetness to this dish, making it perfect if you want to satisfy your strongest sweet tooth.

Makes: 2 Servings

Total Prep Time: 25 Minutes

Ingredients:

- 1 Cup of Brussels Sprouts, Cleaned and Cut into Halves
- ¼ Cup of Olive Oil, Extra Virgin Variety
- 1 Orange, Fresh and Squeezed
- ½ of a Lemon, Freshly Squeezed
- 1 Tbsp. of Pomegranate Molasses
- Dash of Salt, For Taste
- 1 tsp. of Orange, Zest Only
- 3 Tbsp. of Pomegranate Seeds

Directions:

1. First heat up some oil in a large sized skillet place over medium heat. Once the oil is hot enough add in your sprouts and cook for the next three minutes.

2. Pour in your orange and lemon juice into your pan and continue to cook until all of your juice has been evaporated.

3. Add in your pomegranate molasses and reduce the heat to low. Allow your sprouts to caramelize well.

4. Season with some salt and remove from heat.

5. Toss in your remaining ingredients and allow to cool slightly before serving. Enjoy.

Jalapeno and Raspberry Chocolates

If you are a huge fan of delicious chocolate, this is the perfect dish for you. While the different flavors used in this dish make seem unconventional, this is a great tasting dish. I know you are going to love it.

Makes: 12 Servings

Total Prep Time: 20 Minutes

Ingredients:

- 5 Ounces of Chocolate, Dark and Finely Chopped
- ½ of a Jalapeno, Fresh, Seeded and Minced
- 1/3 Cup of Raspberries, Fresh
- 2 Tbsp. of Agave
- Some Chocolate Molds

Directions:

1. In a small sized sauce pan placed over low heat, melt your chocolate until smooth in consistency.

2. Once melted spoon a small amount of your chocolate into a mold. Place into your fridge for the next 5 minutes or until your chocolate has fully set.

3. Next mash your raspberries with your jalapeno and agave until thoroughly mixed.

4. Fill each mold with your raspberry filling and spoon more chocolate over your filling.

5. Place back into your fridge to fill for the next 10 minutes or until completely set.

6. Remove and serve whenever you are ready.

Sugar Free Brownies

If are a huge fan of brownies, then this is the perfect dish for you. These brownies are incredibly healthy for you as they are both grain free and sugar free. I know you won't be able to get enough of them.

Makes: 6 Servings

Total Prep Time: 45 Minutes

Ingredients:

- 4 Ounces of Butter, Soft
- 8 Ounces of Chocolate, Dark in Color
- 1 Tbsp. of Cocoa, Powdered Variety
- 3 Tbsp. of Oil, Avocado Variety
- 1 tsp. of Stevia, Powdered Variety
- 1 tsp. of Baker's Style Baking Powder
- 3 Eggs, Large in Size and Beaten Lightly
- 1/3 Cup of Flour, Almond Variety
- 1 Tbsp. of Flour, Coconut Variety

Directions:

1. The first thing that you will want to do is preheat your oven to 350 degrees.

2. While your oven is heating up butter a medium sized brownie pan with some butter. Set aside for later use.

3. Then place your butter, chocolate and oil into a double boiler. Stir thoroughly until your chocolate and butter are thoroughly melted.

4. Add in your remaining ingredients and stir until thick in consistency.

5. Pour your batter into your prepared brownie dish. Place into your oven to bake for the next 35 minutes or until completely set.

6. Remove and allow to cool slightly before serving. Enjoy.

Valentine's Day Chia Pudding

Here is a vegan style chia pudding dish that I know you are going to love. It is incredibly healthy as it is packed full of antioxidants, protein, omega 3 fatty acids and fiber. You never have to worry about feeling guilty about enjoying this dish.

Makes: 2 Servings

Total Prep Time: 4 to 5 Hours

Ingredients:

- 3 Tbsp. of Chia Seeds
- 1 Cup of Milk, Coconut Variety
- 1 Tbsp. of Agave Nectar
- 1 tsp. of Vanilla, Pure
- 2 Cups of Raspberries, Fresh
- 1 Tbsp. of Coconut Flakes

Directions:

1. First use a medium sized bowl and combine your seeds and coconut milk together until thoroughly combined and smooth in consistency.

2. Then add in your nectar and vanilla and stir thoroughly until combined. Divide your mixture between two medium sized bowls.

3. Cover with some plastic wrap and place into your fridge to chill for the next 4 to 5 hours.

4. After this time puree your raspberries in a food processor until smooth in consistency. Pour into one of your chia seed mixtures.

5. Spoon your mixed raspberry and chia seed mixture into a glass and top off with your other chia seed mixture.

6. Top off with your coconut flakes and enjoy immediately.

Raw Chocolate Pudding

This is a completely raw and sugar free pudding that will help you satisfy your strongest sweet tooth. Even the pickiest of eaters will fall in love with this dish.

Makes: 3 Servings

Total Prep Time: 1 Hour

Ingredients for Your Pudding:

- 3 Bananas, Medium in Size and Peeled
- ½ of an Avocado, Medium in Size and Pitted
- ¼ Cup of Butter, Almond Variety, Smooth in Consistency and Raw
- 4 to 5 Tbsp. of Cacao Powder, Raw and for Taste
- 1 tsp. of Vanilla, Pure
- Dash of Sea Salt, For Taste

Ingredients for Toppings:

- Some Whipped Cream, Coconut Variety
- ¼ Cup of Hazelnuts, Toasted and Finely Chopped

Directions:

1. Add all of your pudding ingredients into a food processor and process until smooth in consistency.

2. Place into your fridge to chill for the next hour.

3. After this time serve with your recommend toppings and enjoy right away.

Chocolate Dipped Mandarin Slices

If you are looking for a healthy and absolutely delicious afternoon snack to enjoy, then this is the perfect dish for you to make. It is the ultimate dish to enjoy if you are looking to satisfy your strongest sweet tooth.

Makes: 5 Servings

Total Prep Time: 20 Minutes

Ingredients:

- 5 Oranges, Mandarin Variety
- ½ Cup of Chocolate Chips, Dark in Color
- Dash of Sea Salt, For Taste
- 1 tsp. of Shortening, Optional

Directions:

1. The first thing that you will want to do is line a baking sheet with some parchment paper and set aside for later use.

2. Then peel your oranges.

3. Then use a microwave safe bowl and melt your chocolate and shortening together until smooth in consistency.

4. Dip each slice of your mandarin halfway into your chocolate and place onto your baking sheet.

5. Sprinkle some salt over the top and place into your fridge to chill for the next 10 minutes or until your chocolate is hard to the touch. Enjoy immediately.

Conclusion

Well, there you have it!

Hopefully by the end of this book you have learned how beneficial aphrodisiacs can be for you, learned about 19 different types of aphrodisiacs you can use to make amazing dishes as well as discovered over 25 of the most delicious aphrodisiac recipes you will ever come across. I hope that by the end of this book you have learned what you can do to boost your libido and bring the romance back into your life.

So, what is the next step for you?

The next step for you to take is to begin making all of the recipes you have discovered in this book. Once you have done that there is nothing left to do but enjoy the benefits of these aphrodisiacs, in both enhanced romance and libido.

Good luck!

Author's Afterthoughts

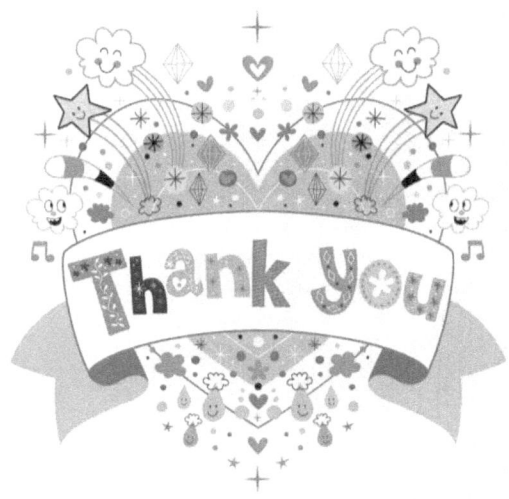

Thanks ever so much to each of my cherished readers for investing the time to read this book!

I know you could have picked from many other books but you chose this one. So a big thanks for downloading this book and reading all the way to the end.

If you enjoyed this book or received value from it, I'd like to ask you for a favor. Please take a few minutes to post an honest and heartfelt review on Amazon.com. Your support does make a difference and helps to benefit other people.

Thanks for your Reviews!

Rachael Rayner

www.ingramcontent.com/pod-product-compliance
Lightning Source LLC
Chambersburg PA
CBHW030519290526
45786CB00004B/1533